Low Carb Casseroles:
25 Satisfying L

MW01108002

Table of content

Introduction

There you are, exciting to start you new diet, and watch that weight fall off. You know you have tried different diets before, and they all seem to work for a while, but you soon get bored on them, and wish that you could have the same foods you have always loved.

Sure, you can have some of the things that you once did, but when you look at the so called substitutes, you know there is no way you are going to stick with it for the long term.

You can't go without your meat, and you can't go without your cheese. You know you are in love with your pastas... but wait... you are now low carb, and that means pasta is off limits!

Or does it?

While you may not get to indulge in the same kind of pasta you once did, you are going to discover that there is something so much better, not only better for you but better tasting, and you won't ever want to go back. Let me show you the secret to enjoying your low carb diet in a way that you can stick with long term, and forget worrying about whether or not this is going to work.

When you see that you can have the same kinds of foods you have always loved, just with a new, low carb twist, you aren't ever going to want to go back to the way you used to do things.

"But how can I still have lasagna or pizza? Aren't those full of carbs?"

"Chicken and dumplings? There's no way!"

"I'm tired of eating the fake foods, I want to eat something that I know I can enjoy!"

If you have ever felt this way, you are not alone. Countless people who diet get stuck with the feeling they are trapped and can't get out. They can't have the foods that they love, and they are going to be stuck on a diet they hate for the rest of their lives.

But this is going to change all of that. I am going to give you the recipes you need to love the diet you are on, and to want to stick with it for the long term.

So if you are ready to break out of the restrictive diet you are on and indulge in the freedom of low carb, you have come to the right place. Enjoy.

Chapter 1 – Fast 'N Easy Low Carb Casseroles

Chicken Nugget Casserole

What you will need:

1 cup almond flour

3 tablespoons butter

Salt

Pepper

3 boneless skinless chicken breasts

1 can cream of chicken soup

1 bag frozen corn

1 bag frozen peas

Directions:

Cut the chicken into bite sized pieces and brown in a pan on the stove. Use a little vegetable oil to keep from burning.

Thaw the bags of veggies in the microwave and drain off the liquid. Mix the can of soup with half a can of milk, then combine all ingredients except the butter and flour in your 9 x 13 inch baking dish.

Melt the butter in a dish in the microwave and cut into the almond flour, then spread over the top of the casserole.

Preheat oven to 350 degrees F.

Place your 9 x 13 inch baking dish covered in foil on the center rack and bake for 15 minutes.

Uncover and bake for another 10 minutes, then pull out of the oven and let sit on a hot pad for an additional 5 minutes. Serve with your favorite low carb side dish.

Serves 4- 6.

"Mac"'n'Cheese Casserole

What you will need:

1 cup coconut flour

1 cup milk

2 tablespoons butter

1 head cauliflower

1 head broccoli

2 packages cheddar cheese

Directions:

Chop the cauliflower into smaller pieces and break the broccoli into smaller pieces. You want the broccoli to be larger than the cauliflower.

Heat the milk on the stove, and combine the butter, milk, and cheese until the cheese is melted. Stir in the coconut flour, followed by the cauliflower.

Stir to coat.

Add in the broccoli, then transfer to your 9 x 13 inch baking dish.

Preheat oven to 350 degrees F.

Place your 9 x 13 inch baking dish covered in foil on the center rack and bake for 15 minutes.

Uncover and bake for another 10 minutes, then pull out of the oven and let sit on a hot pad for an additional 5 minutes. Serve with your favorite low carb side dish.

Serves 4- 6.

Sweeter Than Chili Casserole

What you will need:

2 pounds burger

1 onion

1 package frozen corn

2 tablespoons chili powder

Salt

Pepper

2 cans diced tomatoes

Directions:

Chop the onion and brown with the burger on the stove. Add in the corn until it is thawed, and open the cans of tomatoes.

Do not drain the tomatoes, but do drain the burger. Combine everything in your 9 x 13 inch pan and cover with foil.

Preheat oven to 350 degrees F.

Place your 9 x 13 inch baking dish covered in foil on the center rack and bake for 15 minutes.

Uncover and bake for another 10 minutes, then pull out of the oven and let sit on a hot pad for an additional 5 minutes. Serve with your favorite low carb side dish.

Serves 4- 6.

Corn Cob Casserole

What you will need:

2 packages baby corn cobs

1 head cauliflower

1 package fresh green beans

Salt

Pepper

1 small brick cheddar cheese, cubed

Directions:

Thaw the frozen veggies and drain the excess liquid off of them. Chop the cauliflower and cube the brick of cheese before combining everything in a 9 x 13 inch baking dish.

Preheat oven to 350 degrees F.

Place your 9 x 13 inch baking dish covered in foil on the center rack and bake for 15 minutes.

Uncover and bake for another 10 minutes, then pull out of the oven and let sit on a hot pad for an additional 5 minutes. Serve with your favorite low carb side dish.

Serves 4- 6.

Chicken Pot Pie

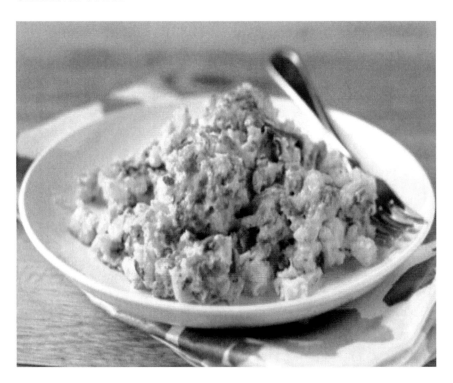

What you will need:

3 boneless skinless chicken breasts

1 cup almond flour

1 can peas

1 can corn

1 egg

1 can cream of chicken soup

1 can full fat coconut cream

Salt

Pepper

Directions:

Cut the chicken into bite sized pieces and brown on the stove. You don't have to cook them fully, but make sure they are at least halfway done.

Open and drain the veggies, and combine in a dish with the coconut cream and soup.

Combine all of these now in a 9 x 13 inch baking pan, spreading them out evenly. In another dish, combine the egg and the flour. Sprinkle this over the rest of the ingredients now, and cover with foil.

Preheat oven to 350 degrees F.

Place your 9 x 13 inch baking dish covered in foil on the center rack and bake for 15 minutes.

Uncover and bake for another 10 minutes, then pull out of the oven and let sit on a hot pad for an additional 5 minutes. Serve with your favorite low carb side dish.

Serves 4- 6.

Cheeseburger Casserole

What you will need:

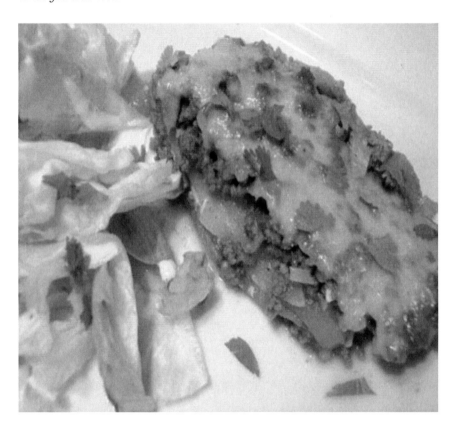

2 pounds burger

Salt

Pepper

1 package bacon

1 package shredded cheese

1 can diced tomatoes

1 package cauliflower

Directions:

Brown the burger on the stove along with the bacon cut into bite sized pieces. Season with salt and pepper. Combine the diced tomatoes with the cauliflower, and spread everything in a 9 x 13 inch baking pan.

Cover with the cheese and foil.

Preheat oven to 350 degrees F.

Place your 9 x 13 inch baking dish covered in foil on the center rack and bake for 15 minutes.

Uncover and bake for another 10 minutes, then pull out of the oven and let sit on a hot pad for an additional 5 minutes. Serve with your favorite low carb side dish.

Serves 4- 6.

BBQ Casserole

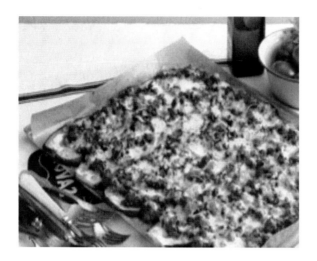

What you will need:

2 pounds pork ribs

1 bottle BBQ sauce

1 package baby corn on the cob

1 package cauliflower

1 green pepper

Salt

Pepper

Directions:

Brown the ribs on the stove top. You don't need to cook them thoroughly, but make sure they have a good start.

Lay them in the 9 x 13 inch baking dish. Spread the cauliflower and baby corn around the ribs, and season with the salt and pepper. Generously pour the BBQ sauce over the top, garnish with the chopped green pepper, and top with foil.

Preheat oven to 350 degrees F.

Place your 9 x 13 inch baking dish covered in foil on the center rack and bake for 15 minutes.

Uncover and bake for another 10 minutes, then pull out of the oven and let sit on a hot pad for an additional 5 minutes. Serve with your favorite low carb side dish.

Serves 4- 6.

Cowboy Casserole

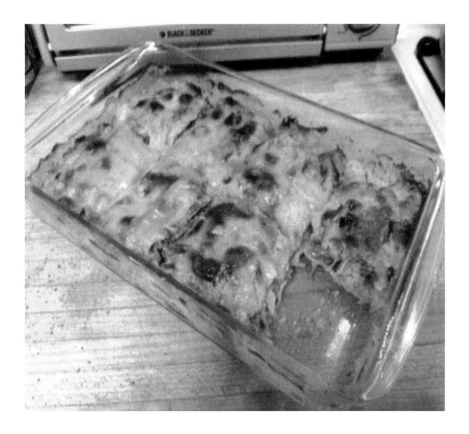

What you will need:

1 pound burger

2 pounds bacon

2 cups almond flour

2 eggs

1 tablespoon water

Salt

Pepper

Cut the bacon into bite sized pieces and brown with the burger on the stove. In a separate dish, combine the eggs with the flour and water, until it is batter like.

Transfer the bacon and burger to a 9 x 13 inch pan, and spread the batter over the top. Garnish with cheese, if desired, and cover with foil.

Preheat oven to 350 degrees F.

Place your 9 x 13 inch baking dish covered in foil on the center rack and bake for 15 minutes.

Uncover and bake for another 10 minutes, then pull out of the oven and let sit on a hot pad for an additional 5 minutes. Serve with your favorite low carb side dish.

Serves 4- 6.

T-Rex Casserole

What you will need:

1 pork roast

1 bottle BBQ Sauce

1 large Zucchini

1 small yellow zucchini

Directions:

Slice the zucchini into discs and cut the cooked pork roast into bite sized pieces. Combine all ingredients in a 9 x 13 inch baking dish, and cover with foil.

Preheat oven to 350 degrees F.

Place your 9 x 13 inch baking dish covered in foil on the center rack and bake for 15 minutes.

Uncover and bake for another 10 minutes, then pull out of the oven and let sit on a hot pad for an additional 5 minutes. Serve with your favorite low carb side dish.

Serves 4- 6.

Jack and Jill Casserole

What you will need:

3 zucchini

1 jar spaghetti sauce

1 can diced tomatoes

2 packages mozzarella cheese

1 package cottage cheese

Salt

Pepper

1 pound burger

Directions:

Brown the burger on the stove with some salt and pepper to taste. As this is browning, cut the zucchini lengthwise into long boats. Carefully slice them once more lengthwise, so you have 2 boats and a middle section.

Place the bottom of the boats on the bottom of your 9 x 13 inch pan. Spread 1/3 of the spaghetti sauce next, plus 1 package mozzarella and ½ of the burger.

Lay down the middle layer of the zucchini. Next add the cottage cheese, then another layer of spaghetti sauce.

Lay the final layer of zucchini, followed by the rest of the sauce, the rest of the burger, and the rest of the cheese. Cover with foil.

Preheat oven to 350 degrees F.

Place your 9 x 13 inch baking dish covered in foil on the center rack and bake for 15 minutes.

Uncover and bake for another 10 minutes, then pull out of the oven and let sit on a hot pad for an additional 5 minutes. Serve with your favorite low carb side dish.

Serves 4- 6.

Breakfast Casserole

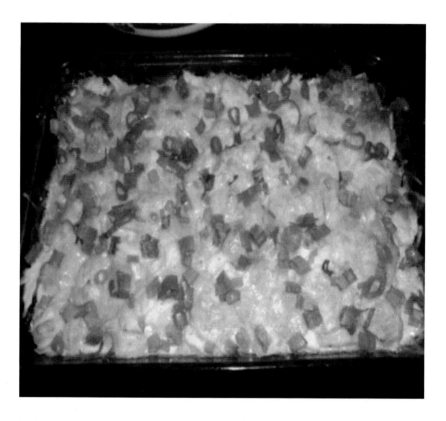

https://www.google.com/search?
q=simple+low+carb+casseroles&espv=2&biw=1366&bih=662&source=lnms&tbm=isch&sa=X&ved=0ahUKEwjBh7Syvt-
HPAhVB1WMKHZVzAjsQ_AUIBygC&dpr=1

What you will need:

6 eggs

1 pound breakfast sausage

1 package cheddar cheese

Salt

Pepper

1 cup milk

3 green peppers

Directions:

Brown the sausage on the stove until cooked thoroughly. Drain and set aside.

Combine the eggs and milk with half the cheddar cheese, and chop the green peppers. Stir these into the mix before adding in the sausage.

Transfer everything into a 9 x 13 inch baking dish and garnish with the rest of the cheese. Garnish with a bit of the pepper before you cover with foil.

Preheat oven to 350 degrees F.

Place your 9 x 13 inch baking dish covered in foil on the center rack and bake for 15 minutes.

Uncover and bake for another 10 minutes, then pull out of the oven and let sit on a hot pad for an additional 5 minutes. Serve with your favorite low carb side dish.

Serves 4- 6.

Chicken Dumplin' Low Carb Style

What you will need:

3 boneless skinless chicken breasts

2 cups coconut flour

3 eggs

1 can cream of chicken soup

1 cup chicken broth

½ cup chopped carrots

1 package cauliflower

Salt

Pepper

Directions:

Cut the chicken into bite sized pieces and place in a pan on the stove. Brown the outside of the chicken but don't cook all the way. Set aside.

Thaw the cauliflower, and drain the excess liquid. Combine the eggs with 1/3 of the chicken broth and all the flour. Form cakes with these and set aside.

Combine all ingredients now except for these cakes in a 9 x 13 inch baking dish. Set these dumplings over the top, and cover with foil.

Preheat oven to 350 degrees F.

Place your 9 x 13 inch baking dish covered in foil on the center rack and bake for 15 minutes.

Uncover and bake for another 10 minutes, then pull out of the oven and let sit on a hot pad for an additional 5 minutes. Serve with your favorite low carb side dish.

Serves 4- 6.

Thanksgiving Casserole

What you will need:

2 pounds turkey burger

1 bag frozen corn

1 bag cranberries

1 can cream of celery soup

1 can milk

2 stalks celery

Salt

Pepper

Directions:

Brown the turkey burger on the stove until cooked thoroughly. Scrub and chop the celery, then combine the soup, celery, salt and pepper. Drain the turkey burger and add to the mix. Thaw the corn and drain the liquid before adding next, then finish with the cranberries.

Spread evenly on the bottom of a 9 x 13 inch baking dish, and cover with foil.

Preheat oven to 350 degrees F.

Place your 9 x 13 inch baking dish covered in foil on the center rack and bake for 15 minutes.

Uncover and bake for another 10 minutes, then pull out of the oven and let sit on a hot pad for an additional 5 minutes. Serve with your favorite low carb side dish.

Serves 4- 6.

Best Ever Broccoli Casserole

What you will need:

2 packages broccoli

1 red pepper

1 green pepper

1 yellow pepper

2 boneless skinless chicken breasts

1 can cream of chicken soup

1 can milk

Salt

Pepper

1 package cheddar cheese

Directions:

Cut the chicken into bite sized pieces and brown on the stove with a bit of vegetable oil.

Slice the peppers and wash thoroughly, then thaw the broccoli and drain the excess liquid. Combine the soup and milk with the pepper and salt, then combine all ingredients in a 9 x 13 inch baking dish.

Garnish with the cheddar cheese and cover with foil.

Preheat oven to 350 degrees F.

Place your 9 x 13 inch baking dish covered in foil on the center rack and bake for 15 minutes.

Uncover and bake for another 10 minutes, then pull out of the oven and let sit on a hot pad for an additional 5 minutes. Serve with your favorite low carb side dish.

Serves 4- 6.

Green Bean Casserole

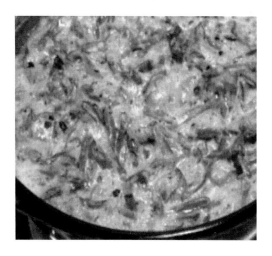

What you will need:

2 cans green beans

2 packages cheddar cheese

1 can cream of mushroom soup

1 carton sour cream

Directions:

Open the cans of green beans and spread them evenly on the bottom of a 9 x 13 inch baking dish. Combine the cream of mushroom soup with the sour cream, and spread over the top of the green beans.

Sprinkle the cheese over the top, and garnish with salt and pepper, if you like. Cover with foil.

Preheat oven to 350 degrees F.

Place your 9 x 13 inch baking dish covered in foil on the center rack and bake for 15 minutes.

Uncover and bake for another 10 minutes, then pull out of the oven and let sit on a hot pad for an additional 5 minutes. Serve with your favorite low carb side dish.

Serves 4- 6.

Sqishity Squash Casserole

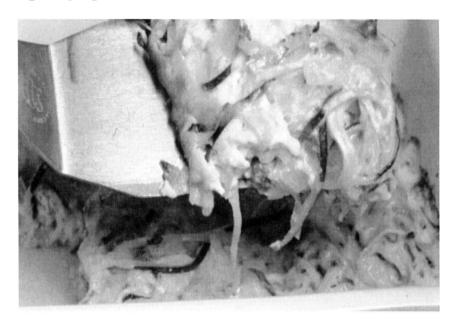

https://www.google.com/search?
q=simple+low+carb+casseroles&espv=2&biw=1366&bih=662&source=lnms&tbm=isch&sa=X&ved=0ahUKEwjBh7Syvt-HPAhVB1WMKHZVzAjsQ_AUIBygC&dpr=1

What you will need:

2 yellow squash

1 package cauliflower

2 tablespoons butter

2 jars cranberry sauce

Directions:

Begin by partially baking the squash in your oven for 10 minutes. You don't want it to be cooked all the way through, but you do want it to be soft.

Scoop out the center and spread across the bottom of a 9 x 13 inch baking dish. Thaw the cauliflower and drain the liquid, then press into the squash.

Cut the butter into the mix, and spread the cranberry sauce over the top before you cover with foil.

Preheat oven to 350 degrees F.

Place your 9 x 13 inch baking dish covered in foil on the center rack and bake for 15 minutes.

Uncover and bake for another 10 minutes, then pull out of the oven and let sit on a hot pad for an additional 5 minutes. Serve with your favorite low carb side dish.

Serves 4- 6.

Fall's Here Pumpkin Casserole

What you will need:

2 packages cauliflower

2 large cans pumpkin

1 can corn

Salt

Pepper

1 can milk

Directions:

Thaw and drain the excess liquid off of the cauliflower before opening the cans of pumpkin. Scoop everything into a 9 x 13 inch pan, and open and drain the can of corn.

Season with garlic, salt, and pepper, and spread evenly on the bottom of the pan, then cover with foil.

Preheat oven to 350 degrees F.

Place your 9 x 13 inch baking dish covered in foil on the center rack and bake for 15 minutes.

Uncover and bake for another 10 minutes, then pull out of the oven and let sit on a hot pad for an additional 5 minutes. Serve with your favorite low carb side dish.

Serves 4- 6.

Eggplant Delight

What you will need:

1 large eggplant

2 pounds breakfast sausage

Salt

Pepper

1 package cheddar cheese

Directions:

Slice the eggplant first lengthwise, then cut it into bite sized pieces. Brown the burger on the stove until it is cooked, then combine both in a 9 x 13 inch baking dish.

Season with the salt and pepper to taste, then sprinkle the shredded cheese over the top. Cover with foil.

Preheat oven to 350 degrees F.

Place your 9 x 13 inch baking dish covered in foil on the center rack and bake for 15 minutes.

Uncover and bake for another 10 minutes, then pull out of the oven and let sit on a hot pad for an additional 5 minutes. Serve with your favorite low carb side dish.

Serves 4- 6.

Good Time Mexican Casserole

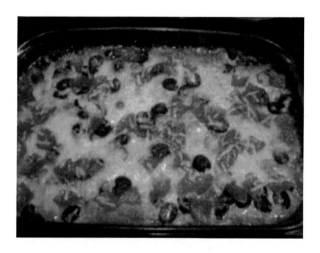

What you will need:

2 pounds burger

2 tablespoons taco seasoning

1 can corn

1 can green chili peppers

1 can olives

1 green pepper

1 carton sour cream

1 can diced tomatoes

1 package shredded cheese

Directions:

Brown the burger on the stove and season with the taco seasoning. Open the cans and drain off all the liquid, then combine all the veggies in a separate dish. Stir the burger in with the veggies, then transfer into a 9 x 13 inch baking dish.

Spread the sour cream over the top, and garnish with the cheese. Cover with foil.

Preheat oven to 350 degrees F.

Place your 9 x 13 inch baking dish covered in foil on the center rack and bake for 15 minutes.

Uncover and bake for another 10 minutes, then pull out of the oven and let sit on a hot pad for an additional 5 minutes. Serve with your favorite low carb side dish.

Serves 4- 6.

Barnyard Casserole

What you will need:

6 eggs

1 package pork sausage

1 package bacon

1 package corn

2 green peppers

1 package cauliflower

Salt

Pepper

1 package cheese

Directions:

Cut the bacon into bite sized pieces, and cook the sausage thoroughly. Thaw the package of cauliflower, and drain off the excess liquid.

Chop the peppers, and combine everything but the cheese with the eggs. Transfer to a 9 x 13 inch baking dish and garnish with the cheese, salt, and pepper.

Cover with foil.

Preheat oven to 350 degrees F.

Place your 9 x 13 inch baking dish covered in foil on the center rack and bake for 15 minutes.

Uncover and bake for another 10 minutes, then pull out of the oven and let sit on a hot pad for an additional 5 minutes. Serve with your favorite low carb side dish.

Serves 4- 6.

Easy Pepperoni Casserole

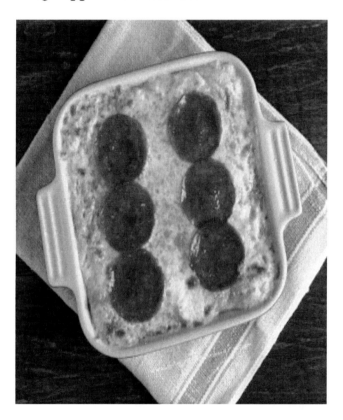

What you will need:

2 packages cauliflower

2 eggs

1 cup almond flour

1 package pepperoni

1 jar tomato sauce

2 packages mozzarella

Directions:

In a food processor, chop the cauliflower as small as you can manage. Combine this with the almond flour and the eggs, then press into the bottom of your 9 x 13 inch casserole baking dish.

Spread the tomato sauce over the top, then the cheese next. Finish with the pepperoni and cover with foil.

Preheat oven to 350 degrees F.

Place your 9 x 13 inch baking dish covered in foil on the center rack and bake for 15 minutes.

Uncover and bake for another 10 minutes, then pull out of the oven and let sit on a hot pad for an additional 5 minutes. Serve with your favorite low carb side dish.

Serves 4- 6.

Green Chicken Casserole

What you will need:

3 boneless skinless chicken breasts

2 green peppers

1 jar alfredo sauce

1 package parmesan cheese

1 onion

1 can green chili peppers

Directions:

Cut the chicken into bite sized pieces and brown on the stove. Wash and cut the green peppers, and chop the onion. Soften the onion in the pan with the chicken.

Open and drain the can of green chili peppers, then combine all ingredients excepts for the parmesan in a 9 x 13 inch baking dish.

Garnish with the parmesan, and cover with foil.

Preheat oven to 350 degrees F.

Place your 9 x 13 inch baking dish covered in foil on the center rack and bake for 15 minutes.

Uncover and bake for another 10 minutes, then pull out of the oven and let sit on a hot pad for an additional 5 minutes. Serve with your favorite low carb side dish.

Serves 4- 6.

The Awesome Asparagus Casserole

What you will need:

2 packages asparagus

1 package green beans

1 package cauliflower

1 package cheddar cheese

1 package parmesan cheese

1 cup almond flour

1 cup milk

1 tablespoon butter

Salt

Pepper

Directions:

Thaw the green beans, cauliflower, and asparagus in the microwave, and drain all the excess liquid. Heat the milk on the stove and melt the butter, then add in the cheese and the flour.

You may have to add in extra milk if it gets too thick.

Combine all ingredients in your 9 x 13 inch baking dish, and cover with foil.

Preheat oven to 350 degrees F.

Place your 9 x 13 inch baking dish covered in foil on the center rack and bake for 15 minutes.

Uncover and bake for another 10 minutes, then pull out of the oven and let sit on a hot pad for an additional 5 minutes. Serve with your favorite low carb side dish.

Serves 4- 6.

Superman Casserole

What you will need:

1 package bacon

1 pound pork sausage

1 pound hamburger

1 eggplant

1 jar tomato sauce

Salt

Pepper

Directions:

Cut the bacon into bite sized pieces and brown with the burger and sausage on the stove. Once completely browned, remove from heat and drain the grease.

Cut the eggplant into bite sized pieces and stir into the mix. Stir in the tomato sauce next, and garnish with cheese, if desired.

Cover with foil.

Preheat oven to 350 degrees F.

Place your 9 x 13 inch baking dish covered in foil on the center rack and bake for 15 minutes.

Uncover and bake for another 10 minutes, then pull out of the oven and let sit on a hot pad for an additional 5 minutes. Serve with your favorite low carb side dish.

Serves 4- 6.

The Mushy Mozzarella Casserole

What you will need:

3 packages mushrooms, either fresh or large cans

2 pounds burger

1 jar diced tomatoes

2 packages mozzarella cheese

Directions:

Brown the burger on the stove with a bit of salt and pepper to taste. Add in the mushrooms and let simmer together for a moment, before draining the liquid.

Open and drain the can of diced tomatoes and add this to the mix. Transfer everything to your 9 x 13 inch baking dish, and cover with the mozzarella cheese. Spread foil over the top.

Preheat oven to 350 degrees F.

Place your 9 x 13 inch baking dish covered in foil on the center rack and bake for 15 minutes.

Uncover and bake for another 10 minutes, then pull out of the oven and let sit on a hot pad for an additional 5 minutes. Serve with your favorite low carb side dish.

Serves 4- 6.

Conclusion

There you have it, everything you need to get out there and enjoy low carb dinners with your friends and family, and to enjoy the same kinds of foods you did before you went low carb.

I know what it's like when you are first trying out any diet. All of a sudden, you want anything and everything that is on the list of foods you aren't supposed to have. Suddenly, you can't imagine life without eating pasta, even if you haven't had pasta in the past few weeks.

Suddenly, all you can think of is the old foods you used to have together, and you think that there's no way you can ever get anyone else on board with what you are eating now. But that's not true, and this book is going to change all of that.

I hope this book was able to show you that you can have low carb foods that everyone can enjoy, and that you can have them with the people you love. There's no need to worry about having to make something different for your company.

With the recipes in this book, you not only can make the same dish for everyone, but everyone is going to enjoy what you make. Soon, you are going to have everyone asking you for what recipes you used, even if your friends and family aren't low carb.

You see, when you are eating a certain way, all you care about is if it's healthy for you, and if you can enjoy it with the people you love. If you can say yes to both of those questions, you know you have a winner. And that is exactly what I wanted to give you with the recipes in this book.

I wanted to give you the freedom to enjoy the diet you are on while you lose weight, and to be able to enjoy it with the people you love. With these recipes, not only are you going to lose the weight you want to lose, but you can take what you learn here and apply them to other recipes for even more variety.

Welcome to the world of loving your diet, and still losing weight.

Dinner is served.

FREE Bonus Reminder

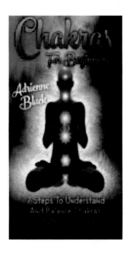

If you have not grabbed it yet, please go ahead and download your special bonus E book *"Chakras for Beginners. 7 Steps To Understand And Balance Chakras, Radiate Energy, And Strengthen Aura"*.

Simply Click the Button Below

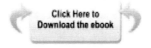

OR Go to This Page

http://lifehacksworld.com/free

BONUS #2: More Free & Discounted Books & Products

Do you want to receive more Free/Discounted Books or Products?

We have a mailing list where we send out our new Books or Products when they go free or with a discount on Amazon. Click on the link below to sign up for Free & Discount Book & Product Promotions.

=> Sign Up for Free & Discount Book & Product Promotions <=

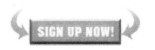

OR Go to this URL

http://zbit.ly/1WBb1Ek

Made in United States
Cleveland, OH
28 May 2025

17310317R00026